Quick and easy complete solution parkinson disease diet cookbook: for beginners

Say No to Parkinson pain, Get ready to practice special delicious 100+recipes magic,+28day meal plan to living longer.

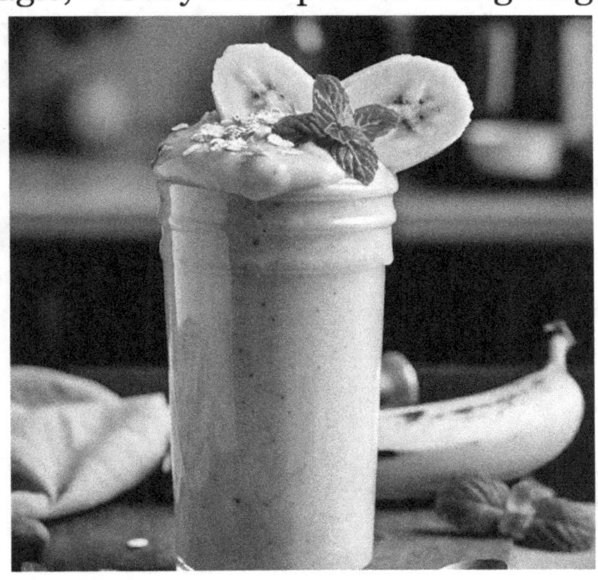

Dr. Jerry Cole

TABLE OF CONTENT

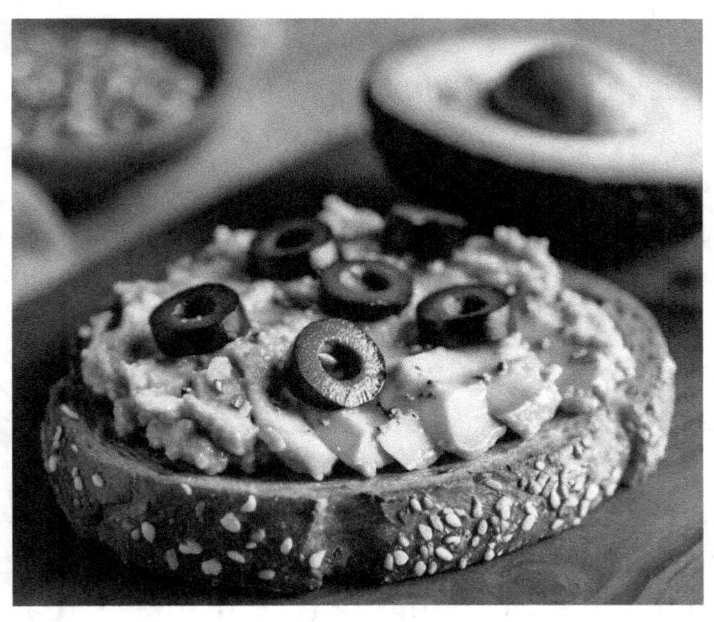

INTRODUCTION

"Welcome to the Quick and Easy Complete Solution Parkinson's Disease Diet Cookbook for Beginners! If you or a loved one has been diagnosed with Parkinson's disease, you know that managing the condition requires a comprehensive approach that includes medication, exercise, and nutrition.

While there is no cure for Parkinson's disease, research has shown that a healthy diet can play a crucial role in alleviating symptoms, slowing disease progression, and improving overall quality of life. But with so much conflicting information out there, it can be overwhelming to know where to start.

That's why we created this cookbook - to provide a simple, easy-to-follow guide to cooking delicious and nutritious meals that support Parkinson's disease management. Our recipes are designed specifically for beginners, with clear instructions and minimal ingredients to get you started right away.

In this cookbook, you'll find:

- 100+ quick and easy recipes tailored to Parkinson's disease dietary needs

- Nutritious and wholesome ingredients to support brain health and overall well-being
- Step-by-step instructions and photos to make cooking a breeze
- Tips and tricks for meal prep, cooking, and nutrition
- A comprehensive guide to understanding Parkinson's disease and the role of nutrition in management

Our goal is to empower you with the knowledge and tools you need to take control of your diet and nutrition, and to make a positive impact on your health and well-being. So let's get cooking, and start feeling the benefits of a healthy Parkinson's disease diet today!"

This introduction aims to:

- Welcome and reassure the reader
- Explain the importance of nutrition in managing Parkinson's disease
- Introduce the cookbook and its benefits

- Preview the content and features of the cookbook
- Encourage the reader to start cooking and taking control of their health

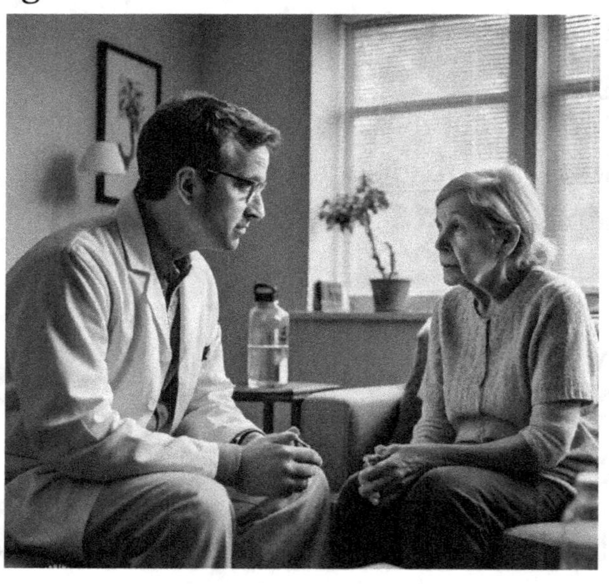

Chapter 1:PARKINSON'S DISEASE: WHAT IS IT?

A degenerative neurological condition that impairs movement is Parkinson's disease. It is brought on by a degeneration of neurons that generate dopamine, a neurotransmitter that aids in the regulation of movement and coordination.

Important details regarding Parkinson's disease:

Tremors, trunk and limb rigidity, bradykinesia, or delayed movement, and problems with balance and coordination are the primary symptoms.

It falls within the movement disorder category. It gets more difficult for the brain to regulate muscle actions as dopamine levels fall.

Although the precise etiology is uncertain, environmental and genetic factors are thought to be involved.

It usually affects those over 60, though it can also strike younger folks.

Levodopa and other dopamine agonists are two drugs that can help control the motor symptoms even though there is no known treatment.

There may also be non-motor symptoms like sadness, difficulty sleeping, and cognitive decline.

Parkinson's disease symptoms worsen with time as more neurons become damaged or die. Everybody progresses at a different rate, though.

Many Parkinson's patients can lead active lives for years with the right care, although the illness can eventually worsen and become more incapacitating.

Chapter 2:THE EFFECT OF DIET ON PARKINSON'S

Further research is necessary to determine whether diet can help control Parkinson's disease symptoms and progression. This is how a person's diet may affect Parkinson's:

Antioxidants: It is thought that oxidative stress, which is linked to the onset of Parkinson's disease, damages brain cells. A diet high in antioxidants from fruits, vegetables, whole grains, and healthy fats may help shield the brain cells from this damage.

Timing of protein: Levodopa, a typical Parkinson's treatment, can be impeded by protein in its absorption. For optimal medication absorption, many individuals are advised to split their protein consumption and levodopa dosing by 30 to 1 hour.

Good fats: Diets high in nuts, salmon, and olive oil may have an anti-inflammatory and neuroprotective effect, making them advantageous for Parkinson's sufferers.

Fiber: Due to reduced digestive motility, bowel motions can be problematic for certain Parkinson's patients. A high-fiber diet may assist manage these movements.

Hydration: Drinking enough water is crucial since Parkinson's disease treatments occasionally result in increased perspiration or urine.

Supplements: Further research is required, although several supplements, such as coenzyme Q10, vitamin D, and probiotics, may be beneficial for people with Parkinson's disease.

Make a copy

Chapter 3:WHAT ARE PARKINSON'S DISEASE'S ADVANTAGES AND DISADVANTAGES?

Since Parkinson's disease is a crippling neurological condition, it is challenging to identify any innate advantages. Nonetheless, the following are some possible benefits and drawbacks that Parkinson's patients could encounter:

Enhanced resilience and self-awareness:

For some people, living with a chronic illness such as Parkinson's can result in heightened self-awareness and personal development.

Improved relationships:

Parkinson's disease can strengthen ties between family members and friends, creating stronger support networks.

Motivating lifestyle changes:

A balanced diet, frequent exercise, stress management, and other healthy lifestyle practices can all improve general well-being and may be encouraged by a diagnosis.

DRAWBACKS:

Motor symptoms:

The main drawback of Parkinson's is the gradual loss of motor function, which can greatly affect everyday activities and quality of life. These symptoms include tremors, stiffness, slowness of movement, and balance issues.

Non-motor symptoms:

To make matters more difficult, Parkinson's disease can also result in non-motor symptoms like sadness, cognitive decline, sleep difficulties, and gastrointestinal issues. adverse effects of medication: Dyskinesia (involuntary movements), nausea, and dizziness are common adverse effects of medications used to treat Parkinson's disease symptoms.

For individuals and families, the expense of medical care, therapies, and possible long-term care can be extremely taxing.
Impact on social and emotional aspects: Parkinson's disease can cause social distancing, loss of independence, and emotional discomfort due to its physical and cognitive limits.

As Parkinson's disease advances, the demands of providing day-to-day care for a loved one with the disease can cause physical, mental, and financial stress in caregivers—many of whom are family members.

Chapter 4:PARKINSON'S SYMPTOMS AND CAUSES

PARKINSON'S DISEASE SYMPTOMS:

Motor Signs and Symptoms

Tremor:

a trembling or shaking sensation that usually begins in one hand, arm, or leg. Bradykinesia: Slowness of movement and trouble moving at all.

Rigidity:

The muscles, trunk, and limbs' rigidity or inflexibility.

Postural instability:

Reduced coordination and balance, which raises the possibility of falls.

Freezing:

The momentary incapacity to walk or move. Symptoms Unrelated to the Motor:

Cognitive impairment refers to issues related to memory, focus, and making decisions.

Sleep difficulties include REM sleep behavior disorder, excessive daytime sleepiness, and insomnia.

Mood disorders:

Apathy, depression, and anxiety are prevalent.

Sensory alterations include discomfort, visual issues, and loss of smell.

Constipation, nausea, or difficulty swallowing are examples of digestive disorders.

PARKINSON'S DISEASE CAUSES INCLUDE:

Dopamine deficiency:

The main cause of Parkinson's disease is the death of dopamine-producing neurons in the brain's substantia nigra. One neurotransmitter that is essential for controlling movement is dopamine.

Genetic factors:

Parkinson's disease can arise as a result of mutations in a few genes, including SNCA, LRRK2, and GBA. This is particularly true in patients with an early beginning.

Environmental factors:

Although the precise environmental origins of Parkinson's disease are not well understood, exposure to certain poisons or pesticides, head injuries, and inflammatory processes may raise the risk of the disease.

Lewy bodies:

Parkinson's patients' brain cells produce aberrant protein deposits known as Lewy bodies. It is thought that these protein aggregates play a role in neurodegeneration and cell death.

Oxidative stress:

Over time, oxidative stress can cause damage to neurons in the brain due to an imbalance between antioxidants and free radicals in the brain cells.

Mitochondrial dysfunction:

Individuals with Parkinson's disease may have dysfunctional mitochondria, which results in oxidative stress and a reduction in cellular energy. Mitochondria are the powerhouses of cells.

Although the precise causes of Parkinson's disease are unknown, a hereditary and environmental cocktail is thought to be responsible for the disease's progressive loss of dopamine-producing brain neurons.

Chapter 5: PAIN SOLUTION FOR PARKINSON'S ILLNESS

Parkinson's disease cannot be cured, but there are a number of therapies and coping mechanisms that can help lessen the symptoms, including discomfort. Following are a few methods for treating pain in Parkinson's disease patients:

Levodopa and dopamine agonists are the main drugs used to treat Parkinson's motor symptoms. By increasing movement and lowering muscle stiffness, these drugs can also help with pain reduction in an indirect manner.

NSAIDs, or nonsteroidal anti-inflammatory drugs: NSAIDs, such as ibuprofen or naproxen, are available over-the-counter or on prescription to treat pain and inflammation.

Opioid analgesics: Codeine and tramadol are examples of opioid analgesics that may be administered for severe pain, but they come with a risk of addiction and side effects.

Exercise and physical therapy: Range-of-motion and stretching exercises can assist preserve flexibility and lessen soreness and tightness in the muscles.

Walking and swimming are examples of low-impact aerobic exercises that can increase general strength and mobility while also subtly lowering discomfort.

supplementary treatments

Massage therapy: Can aid in improving circulation and relaxing stiff muscles, which can temporarily relieve discomfort.

Acupuncture: Although its efficacy is still up for question, some Parkinson's patients claim that acupuncture relieves their suffering.

Meditation and mindfulness can enhance coping skills and assist manage stress, which may have an indirect impact on how painful something feels.

Heat and cold therapy: Warm baths or the application of heat pads can help ease pain and stiffness in the muscles.

For the purpose of numbing acute pain and decreasing inflammation, cold packs or ice therapy may be helpful.

Surgical procedures:

Deep brain stimulation (DBS): This surgical technique can aid with pain management and motor complaints by inserting electrodes in the brain to control aberrant neural activity.

Lifestyle changes: Reducing stress, sleeping sufficiently, and keeping a healthy weight can all help with pain management. Indirectly lowering pain, assistive technology such as walkers and canes can enhance mobility and lessen strain.

Chapter 6:FOODS TO AVOID IN PARKINSON'S ILLNESS

People who have Parkinson's disease may want to restrict or stay away from certain foods because they may worsen symptoms, interfere with the absorption of medicines, or present other health risks. The following foods are typically advised to be limited or avoided by people with Parkinson's disease:

Protein-rich foods: Levodopa, a drug that is frequently used for Parkinson's disease, can be absorbed more slowly when consumed with high-protein foods including meat, fish, eggs, cheese, and nuts. It is advised to give yourself at least 30 to 1 hour's break between levodopa doses and the consumption of foods high in protein.

Foods that have been aged, fermented, or **smoked:** Foods with high tyramine content, such as aged cheeses, smoked meats, and fermented foods like pickles and soy sauce, can interact with some Parkinson's drugs and raise blood pressure.

Fried and processed foods: These foods frequently include high levels of sodium, bad fats, and additives, all of which can exacerbate inflammation and other health problems.

Alcohol: Drinking alcohol can make symptoms like tremors and cognitive impairment worse and interfere with some Parkinson's treatments.

While a modest amount of caffeine is generally regarded as harmless, a high amount of caffeine can exacerbate tremors and cause sleep disturbances in certain Parkinson's patients.

Foods high in cholesterol and saturated fat: These include red meat, fried foods, and full-fat dairy products. People with Parkinson's disease are already more likely to develop heart disease and other health issues as a result of these foods.

Foods that dehydrate: Diuretic or high-sodium foods, such coffee, alcohol, and processed snacks, can cause dehydration, which exacerbates symptoms of Parkinson's disease, including constipation.

Chapter 7:FOODS TO INCLUDE FOR PARKINSON'S DISEASE

The following foods are frequently suggested for people with Parkinson's disease:

Foods strong in antioxidants, such as nuts, berries, cherries, leafy greens, and tomatoes, may help shield brain cells from oxidative stress, which is believed to be a factor in the development of Parkinson's disease.

Foods high in fiber: Whole grains, fruits, vegetables, legumes, and other plants are good sources of fiber that can help control bowel movements and ward off constipation, a typical problem in Parkinson's patients.

Omega-3 fatty acids: Rich in omega-3 fatty acids, foods like walnuts, flaxseeds, and fatty fish (salmon, mackerel, and sardines) may have neuroprotective and anti-inflammatory effects.

Probiotics: The gut microbiome can be supported by probiotic-rich foods like yogurt, kefir, and sauerkraut, which may also help relieve the digestive problems that are frequently associated with Parkinson's disease.

Lean proteins: Lean protein sources, like chicken, eggs, and low-fat dairy products, can be consumed in moderation. However, they should be timed correctly to prevent affecting the body's ability to absorb levodopa medicine.

Fluid replacement: It's critical for Parkinson's patients to maintain proper hydration, so sipping water, herbal teas, and low-sugar drinks can help ward off dehydration and constipation.

Foods high in nutrients: Foods high in vitamins and minerals, like fruits, legumes, and leafy greens, can help guarantee a sufficient intake of nutrients, which is crucial for maintaining general health and controlling Parkinson's symptoms.

Chapter 8: THE PARKINSON'S DIET BASICS

Eating for Brain Health

Maintaining general cognitive function and controlling Parkinson's disease may both benefit from eating a diet high in nutrients for the brain. The following dietary advice can help maintain brain function in Parkinson's patients:

Boost your consumption of antioxidants:
These compounds shield brain tissue from oxidative stress, which has been linked to the development of Parkinson's disease. Berries, leafy greens, nuts, and vibrant veggies are good sources.

Pay attention to good fats: Flaxseeds, walnuts, and fatty fish like salmon are good sources of omega-3 fatty acids, which have anti-inflammatory qualities and may help maintain brain function.

Go for whole grains: Fiber, vitamins, and minerals included in whole grains can support gut health, which is connected to brain health, as well as brain performance.

Add some lean proteins: The amino acids required for brain function and the synthesis of neurotransmitters are found in lean proteins such as fish, chicken, lentils, and low-fat dairy products.

Remain hydrated: Drinking enough water can help avoid constipation, which is a common problem in Parkinson's patients, and is essential for cognitive function.

Reduce your intake of processed foods and saturated fats because they can exacerbate oxidative stress and inflammation, which can worsen neurodegeneration.

Think about probiotics: New research indicates that Parkinson's disease may be influenced by gut health, and the probiotics in fermented foods like kefir and yogurt may help maintain a balanced gut microbiota.

Moderate alcohol and caffeine consumption:

While moderate alcohol and caffeine use may improve cognitive function, excessive alcohol and caffeine consumption can impair sleep and lead to dehydration, which can exacerbate Parkinson's symptoms.

Anti-Inflammatory Foods

Since inflammation is believed to contribute to the development of Parkinson's disease, including anti-inflammatory foods in the diet may be advantageous for those who have this neurodegenerative condition. The following foods are suggested as anti-inflammatory for people with Parkinson's disease:

Fatty fish: Omega-3 fatty acids, which are abundant in salmon, mackerel, sardines, and other fatty fish, have strong anti-inflammatory effects.

Extra virgin olive oil: Rich in antioxidants including oleocanthal, which has ibuprofen-like anti-inflammatory properties, and monounsaturated fats, olive oil is a rich source of both.

Leafy greens: Rich in carotenoids, vitamin C, and other antioxidants and anti-inflammatory substances, spinach, kale, and other leafy greens are a great source of health benefits.

Berries: Anthocyanins, which are powerful antioxidant and anti-inflammatory substances, are abundant in blueberries, raspberries, and other berries.

Nuts and seeds: Rich in antioxidants and omega-3 fatty acids that reduce inflammation are almonds, walnuts, chia seeds, and flaxseeds.

Turmeric: Packed with potent anti-inflammatory curcumin, this colorful spice may help shield brain tissue.

Green tea: Green tea has many anti-inflammatory qualities and is high in polyphenol antioxidants, especially epigallocatechin gallate (EGCG).

Tomatoes: Rich in lycopene, an anti-inflammatory antioxidant, tomatoes are a great source of this nutrient.

Garlic and ginger: These tasty ingredients include anti-inflammatory properties including allicin and gingerol.

Fermented foods: Probiotics found in yogurt, kefir, sauerkraut, and other fermented foods can improve gut health and lower inflammation.

Antioxidant-Rich Foods

Antioxidants are substances that have the ability to counteract free radicals and lessen oxidative stress, both of which are believed to be important in the onset and course of Parkinson's disease. Consuming a diet high in antioxidant-rich foods may help shield brain tissue and maybe halt the disease's progression. The following foods high in antioxidants are suggested for Parkinson's patients:

Berries: Antioxidants such as anthocyanins, vitamins C and E, and manganese are abundant in berries, including blueberries, raspberries, strawberries, and other berries.

Leafy greens: Rich in lutein, zeaxanthin, and vitamin C, spinach, kale, and other dark leafy greens are great sources of antioxidants.

Nuts and seeds: Plant components called polyphenols and antioxidants like vitamin E and selenium can be found in abundance in walnuts, almonds, chia seeds, and flaxseeds.

Tomatoes: Rich in lycopene, a potent antioxidant that gives tomatoes their red hue, tomatoes are a great source of this compound.

Lentils and beans: These legumes are rich in minerals like zinc and manganese as well as antioxidants like flavonoids and polyphenols.

Herbs and spices: Antioxidant components such as rosmarinic acid, curcumin, and cinnamon are abundant in turmeric, basil, oregano, and cinnamon.

Dark chocolate: Packed with flavanols, a kind of antioxidant that may enhance cognitive performance, dark chocolate has a high cocoa content.

Epigallocatechin gallate (EGCG), a type of polyphenol antioxidant, is abundant in green tea.

Citrus fruits: Vitamin C, a powerful antioxidant, is abundant in oranges, grapefruits, and other citrus fruits.

Beets: Beets get their vivid color from antioxidant pigments called betalains, which are abundant in beets.

Importance of Fiber

For a number of reasons, fiber is crucial to the nutritional control of Parkinson's disease.

Relieving constipation: One of the most prevalent non-motor symptoms of Parkinson's disease is constipation, which can be brought on by a medication's side effects or delayed digestive motility. By giving the stool more volume and encouraging regular bowel movements, a high-fiber diet can help control bowel motions and stave off constipation.

Gut health: New research points to a possible connection between Parkinson's disease development and gut health. Fiber supports a better gut environment by feeding the good bacteria in the gut microbiome.

Blood sugar control: A significant number of Parkinson's patients either already have type 2 diabetes or are at risk of getting it. Fiber can aid in improving blood sugar regulation by reducing the rate at which glucose enters the bloodstream.

Weight control: For certain people, taking Parkinson's medication and having less movement might lead to weight gain. Foods high in fiber have a tendency to be more satisfying and can increase feelings of fullness, both of which can help you maintain a healthy weight.

Nutrient absorption: Fiber has the ability to slow down the absorption of some nutrients, which may be advantageous for Parkinson's patients who require protein to be taken separately from levodopa medication in order to enhance absorption.

For those with Parkinson's disease, good sources of fiber include:

Whole grains: whole-wheat bread, quinoa, and brown rice

Fruits (apples, pears, berries)

veggies (carrots, broccoli, and Brussels sprouts)

Legumes: black beans, chickpeas, and lentils

Nuts and seeds, such as almonds, flaxseeds, and chia seeds

Drink plenty of water and gradually increase your consumption of fiber to avoid pain or potential bowel blockages.

Managing Protein

For those with Parkinson's disease, controlling protein consumption is crucial since it can impact the effectiveness and absorption of levodopa, a drug that is frequently administered to treat the symptoms of the condition.

Several approaches to controlling protein consumption in Parkinson's disease include:

Protein redistribution: Low protein intake improves levodopa absorption. After taking the final dose of levodopa for the day, the majority of healthcare professionals advise getting most of your protein from food later in the day. This makes it possible for levodopa to be absorbed more effectively both in the morning and during the day.

Levodopa and protein separation: It is advised to give yourself at least 30 to 1 hour's gap between taking levodopa doses and consuming high-protein foods.

Levodopa absorption may be hampered by eating high-protein meals too soon after taking the medication.

Selecting lean protein sources: Lean protein sources include fish, chicken, tofu, lentils, and low-fat dairy products. These are the greatest options when ingesting protein. Compared to high-fat protein sources like red meat, these are typically easier to digest and have less fat.

Monitoring protein intake: Using apps or food diaries to keep track of protein consumption can assist make sure that it is consumed at the right times and in the right amounts in relation to levodopa dosage.

Speaking with a nutritionist: A personalized meal plan that balances protein consumption with other dietary requirements and medication schedules can be created with the assistance of a qualified dietitian.

Staying Hydrated

People with Parkinson's disease need to drink enough water for a number of reasons.

adverse effects of medication: Levodopa and other Parkinson's drugs can produce drooling or excessive perspiration, which can result in dehydration if fluid intake is inadequate.

Handling constipation: One of the most prevalent non-motor symptoms of Parkinson's disease, constipation can get worse due to dehydration. Regular bowel movements and softened stool are encouraged by consuming adequate drinks.

Cognitive function: Cognitive function can be affected by dehydration, which can exacerbate the cognitive symptoms that some Parkinson's patients face.

Orthostatic hypotension: A dip in blood pressure that occurs when standing up and can cause dizziness and fainting is something that Parkinson's disease can exacerbate. Maintaining hydration can lessen this risk.

Dysphagia, or difficulty swallowing, is a potential side effect of Parkinson's disease progression that makes it more difficult for affected individuals to get adequate fluids in their diet. Thicker drinks or foods high in fluids could be advised in certain circumstances.

People with Parkinson's disease should try to drink water frequently throughout the day and eat meals high in fluids, such as fruits, vegetables, and soups, to stay hydrated. Although it's generally advised to consume at least 8 cups (64 ounces) of fluids daily, each person's requirements may differ depending on their age, activity level, and climate.

Other hydrating drinks that can be consumed in addition to water are:

teas made with herbs
fruit-flavored water
reduced-fat milk
diluted fruit juices

It's crucial to minimize or stay away from drinks like alcohol, caffeinated drinks, and sugary sodas that might cause dehydration.

Creating a Balanced Plate

Making a plate that is balanced is a crucial component of a healthy diet for those with Parkinson's disease. You can make sure you're getting the nutrients you need to control symptoms and promote general health by using a balanced plate. These pointers will help you make a plate that is balanced:

Arrange non-starchy vegetables to cover half of the plate:
leafy vegetables (collards, kale, and spinach)
Cruciferous vegetables, such as Brussels sprouts, cauliflower, and broccoli
colorful vegetables (carrots, tomatoes, and bell peppers)

These offer important minerals, fiber, and antioxidants.

Add whole grains to one-quarter of the plate:

Whole-wheat pasta, quinoa, and brown rice

These include B vitamins, fiber, and long-lasting energy.

Add lean protein to one-quarter of the plate:

Fish, poultry, lentils, beans, and tofu

Levodopa can be taken with lean protein sources at the right time since they are easier to digest.

Add a supply of wholesome fats:

Nuts, seeds, avocado, and olive oil

Good fats promote mental wellness and have anti-inflammatory properties.

Include a tiny amount of fruit:

Apples, citrus fruits, and berries

Fruits offer natural sweetness, fiber, and antioxidants.

Remain hydrated:

After every meal, sip on some water, herbal tea, or other beverage.

Good hydration promotes regular bowel movements and the absorption of medications.

Think about serving sizes:

To help with portion management, use smaller plates, particularly for items higher in calories.

By using the balanced plate method, you may control your protein intake, improve your general health, and manage your Parkinson's disease while making sure you're getting a range of nutrients from various food categories.

Chapter 9:STARTING OUT FOR NEWCOMERS TO PARKINSON'S DISEASE

It can be overwhelming for someone who has just received a Parkinson's disease diagnosis to adjust their lifestyle. The following advice can assist newcomers in beginning to control their condition with food and other health-promoting behaviors:

Learn about the importance that nutrition plays in managing Parkinson's disease.

Make sure your diet is well-balanced and full of whole grains, fruits, vegetables, lean proteins, and whole grains.

Recognize how crucial it is to plan your protein consumption around your prescription regimen.

Begin cautiously:
Don't attempt to change your diet drastically all at once. Make gradual, healthful changes.

Start by increasing the amount of fruits, veggies, and whole grains that you eat.

Try out different recipes and cooking techniques that suit your dietary requirements.

Remain hydrated:
Make a conscious effort to increase your daily intake of fluids, especially water.

Keep a water bottle close at hand and make a habit of drinking it.

Prepare in advance: Organizing and preparing your meals can help guarantee that you always have wholesome selections on hand.

If you plan to prepare additional servings, you will have leftovers for busy days.

Seek expert advice: Speak with a qualified nutritionist with experience in Parkinson's disease.

They can create a customized food plan based on your unique requirements and tastes.

Examine your alternatives for exercise: Exercise on a regular basis can help control Parkinson's symptoms and enhance general health.

Begin with easy workouts in a chair or with walking or stretching.

If you have Parkinson's, think about attending a support group or exercise class.

Put self-care first:

Make time for activities that will help you decompress because managing a chronic ailment can be stressful.

Take up hobbies, learn calming techniques, and obtain adequate sleep.

Create a network of support:

Be in the company of loved ones who can support you and who are aware of your situation.

Become a member of a Parkinson's support group to meet people going through similar things.

Recall that altering one's lifestyle requires patience and time. Recognize little accomplishments and don't let losses depress you. You may actively manage your Parkinson's disease with nutrition and healthy behaviors if you have the correct attitude and support.

Chapter 10: COOKING FOR NOVICES WITH PARKINSON'S DISEASE

Cooking can be difficult for people with Parkinson's disease to begin with, but with the correct techniques and equipment, it can be a pleasurable and manageable activity. **Here are some pointers for novices with Parkinson's disease who wish to cook:**

Start with easy recipes: Seek out dishes that only require a few ingredients and clear directions. Choose one-pot dishes, recipes for slow cookers, or basic baking or grilling methods.

Get ready ahead of time: When you have the energy, chop the vegetables, measure the ingredients, and complete as much of the prep work ahead of time. This will simplify and lessen the strain of cooking.

Employ adaptable equipment: To lessen tension and simplify duties, think about using appliances like food choppers, jar openers, electric can openers, and lightweight cookware.

While cooking, take a seat: Make sure you have a cozy place to sit while chopping, blending, or cooking. This may lessen tiredness and help save energy.

Make leftovers a priority: Cook in bulk and store leftovers in the fridge or freezer for simple reheating on days when you're not feeling cooking.

Remain organized: To cut down on distractions and lower the chance of mishaps or falls, keep your kitchen tidy and orderly.

Ask for help: When you need help with grocery shopping, dinner preparation, or cleanup, don't be afraid to ask friends or family for assistance.

Put an emphasis on nutrient-dense foods: To promote general health, include nutrient-dense foods in your meals, such as lean meats, fruits, vegetables, whole grains, and healthy fats.

Control your protein intake: To guarantee the best possible absorption, keep protein-rich meals and levodopa drug doses apart.

Remain hydrated: To stay well-hydrated during cooking, always have water or other hydrating drinks handy.

Put safety first: When handling hot surfaces, sharp objects, and other possible dangers, exercise extreme caution. Use oven mitts or pot holders, and think about using non-slip shoes.

Recall that cooking may be a healing hobby that fosters self-reliance and a feeling of achievement. Notwithstanding the difficulties posed by Parkinson's disease, cooking can be enjoyed with perseverance, imagination, and the appropriate equipment.

Chapter 11: BREAKFAST RECIPES

Banana Oatmeal Smoothie:

- Ingredients:
    1. 1 ripe banana

2. 1/2 cup oats (rolled or quick)
3. 1 cup milk (or almond milk for a dairy-free option)
4. 1 tablespoon honey or maple syrup (optional)
- Instructions:
    1. Peel the banana and break it into chunks.
    2. Place banana chunks, oats, milk, and honey or maple syrup (if using) into a blender.
    3. Blend until smooth and creamy.
    4. Pour into a glass and enjoy immediately.

Scrambled Eggs with Spinach:
- Ingredients:
    1. 2 eggs
    2. 1 cup fresh spinach leaves
    3. Salt and pepper to taste

4. 1 teaspoon olive oil or butter

- Instructions:
    1. Heat olive oil or butter in a non-stick skillet over medium heat.
    2. Add spinach leaves and sauté until wilted.
    3. Crack eggs into the skillet and scramble them with the spinach.
    4. Season with salt and pepper to taste.
    5. Cook until eggs are fully scrambled and cooked through.
    6. Serve hot with whole grain toast or as desired.

Greek Yogurt Parfait:

- Ingredients:
    1. 1/2 cup Greek yogurt
    2. 1/4 cup granola (choose a low-sugar option)

3. 1/2 cup mixed berries (such as strawberries, blueberries, raspberries)
4. 1 tablespoon honey (optional)

- Instructions:
    1. In a glass or bowl, layer Greek yogurt, granola, and mixed berries.
    2. Drizzle honey over the top if desired.
    3. Repeat the layers until ingredients are used up.
    4. Serve immediately as a nutritious and satisfying breakfast.

Whole Grain Toast with Avocado:

- Ingredients:
    1. 2 slices whole grain bread
    2. 1 ripe avocado
    3. Salt and pepper to taste

4. Optional toppings: sliced tomatoes, feta cheese, or red pepper flakes

- Instructions:
    1. Toast the whole grain bread until golden brown.
    2. While the bread is toasting, peel and pit the avocado.
    3. Mash the avocado in a bowl and season with salt and pepper.
    4. Spread mashed avocado evenly onto the toasted bread slices.
    5. Add any desired toppings such as sliced tomatoes, crumbled feta cheese, or red pepper flakes.
    6. Serve immediately for a delicious and nutritious breakfast.

Cottage Cheese with Fruit:

- Ingredients:
  1. 1/2 cup cottage cheese
  2. 1/2 cup mixed fruit (such as pineapple chunks, grapes, and kiwi)
  3. 1 tablespoon chopped nuts (such as almonds or walnuts)
  4. Optional: drizzle of honey or sprinkle of cinnamon
- Instructions:
  1. Spoon cottage cheese into a bowl.
  2. Top with mixed fruit and chopped nuts.
  3. Drizzle with honey or sprinkle with cinnamon if desired.
  4. Serve chilled for a refreshing and protein-packed breakfast option.

Apple Cinnamon Overnight Oats:

- o Ingredients:
    1. 1/2 cup rolled oats
    2. 1/2 cup milk (or almond milk)
    3. 1/2 cup Greek yogurt
    4. 1/2 apple, diced
    5. 1 tablespoon honey or maple syrup
    6. 1/2 teaspoon cinnamon
- o Instructions:
    1. In a mason jar or bowl, combine rolled oats, milk, Greek yogurt, diced apple, honey or maple syrup, and cinnamon.
    2. Stir well to combine.
    3. Cover and refrigerate overnight.
    4. In the morning, give it a stir and enjoy cold or warmed up in the microwave.

Vegetable Egg Muffins:

- Ingredients:
  1. 4 eggs
  2. 1/4 cup diced bell peppers
  3. 1/4 cup diced tomatoes
  4. 1/4 cup diced mushrooms
  5. Salt and pepper to taste
  6. Optional: shredded cheese
- Instructions:
  1. Preheat oven to 350°F (175°C) and grease a muffin tin.
  2. In a bowl, whisk together eggs, diced bell peppers, tomatoes, mushrooms, salt, and pepper.
  3. Pour the egg mixture evenly into the muffin tin, filling each cup about 3/4 full.
  4. If desired, sprinkle shredded cheese on top.

5. Bake for 20-25 minutes or until eggs are set and muffins are golden brown.
6. Allow to cool slightly before serving.

Peanut Butter Banana Toast:

- Ingredients:
    1. 2 slices whole grain bread
    2. 2 tablespoons peanut butter
    3. 1 banana, sliced
    4. Optional: drizzle of honey or sprinkle of cinnamon
- Instructions:
    1. Toast the whole grain bread until golden brown.
    2. Spread peanut butter evenly onto the toasted bread slices.
    3. Arrange sliced banana on top of the peanut butter.

4. Drizzle with honey or sprinkle with cinnamon if desired.

5. Serve immediately for a delicious and energizing breakfast.

Berry Protein Smoothie Bowl:

- Ingredients:
    1. 1 cup mixed berries (such as strawberries, blueberries, raspberries)
    2. 1/2 cup Greek yogurt
    3. 1/4 cup milk (or almond milk)
    4. 1 scoop protein powder (vanilla or berry flavor)
    5. Toppings: sliced almonds, chia seeds, shredded coconut
- Instructions:
    1. In a blender, combine mixed berries, Greek

yogurt, milk, and protein powder.

2. Blend until smooth and creamy.
3. Pour the smoothie into a bowl.
4. Top with sliced almonds, chia seeds, and shredded coconut.
5. Enjoy with a spoon for a nutritious and filling breakfast.

Quinoa Breakfast Bowl:

- Ingredients:
    1. 1/2 cup cooked quinoa
    2. 1/2 cup Greek yogurt
    3. 1/4 cup mixed nuts and seeds (such as almonds, walnuts, pumpkin seeds)
    4. 1/4 cup mixed fresh fruit (such as berries, sliced banana)

5. Optional: drizzle of honey
   or sprinkle of cinnamon
- Instructions:
   1. In a bowl, layer cooked
      quinoa, Greek yogurt,
      mixed nuts and seeds, and
      fresh fruit.
   2. Drizzle with honey or
      sprinkle with cinnamon if
      desired.
   3. Serve immediately for a
      protein-rich and satisfying
      breakfast option.

Chapter 12:LUNCH RECIPES

Vegetable Quinoa Salad:
- Ingredients:
   1. 1/2 cup quinoa
   2. 1 cup water or vegetable
      broth
   3. 1 cup mixed vegetables
      (such as bell peppers,

cucumbers, cherry
tomatoes)

4. 2 tablespoons olive oil
5. 1 tablespoon lemon juice
6. Salt and pepper to taste

- Instructions:
    1. Rinse the quinoa under cold water. In a saucepan, combine quinoa and water or vegetable broth. Bring to a boil, then reduce heat, cover, and simmer for 15 minutes, or until quinoa is cooked and water is absorbed.
    2. In a large bowl, combine cooked quinoa and mixed vegetables.
    3. In a small bowl, whisk together olive oil, lemon juice, salt, and pepper to make the dressing.

4. Pour the dressing over the quinoa and vegetables. Toss until well combined.

5. Serve chilled or at room temperature as a refreshing and nutritious lunch option.

Grilled Chicken Wrap:

- Ingredients:
    1. 1 boneless, skinless chicken breast
    2. 1 whole grain tortilla wrap
    3. 1/4 cup shredded lettuce
    4. 1/4 cup diced tomatoes
    5. 2 tablespoons hummus or Greek yogurt spread
    6. Optional: sliced avocado, shredded cheese
- Instructions:
    1. Season the chicken breast with salt and pepper. Grill or cook in a skillet over medium heat until cooked

through, about 6-8 minutes per side.
2. Slice the cooked chicken breast into thin strips.
3. Lay the tortilla wrap flat and spread hummus or Greek yogurt evenly over it.
4. Place shredded lettuce, diced tomatoes, sliced chicken breast, and any optional ingredients (such as avocado or cheese) onto the wrap.
5. Roll up the wrap tightly, folding in the sides as you go.
6. Cut the wrap in half diagonally and serve immediately, or wrap in foil for an on-the-go lunch.

Mediterranean Chickpea Salad:

- Ingredients:

1. 1 can (15 oz) chickpeas, drained and rinsed
2. 1/2 cucumber, diced
3. 1/2 cup cherry tomatoes, halved
4. 1/4 cup diced red onion
5. 2 tablespoons chopped fresh parsley
6. 2 tablespoons olive oil
7. 1 tablespoon lemon juice
8. Salt and pepper to taste

- Instructions:
  1. In a large bowl, combine chickpeas, cucumber, cherry tomatoes, red onion, and parsley.
  2. In a small bowl, whisk together olive oil, lemon juice, salt, and pepper to make the dressing.
  3. Pour the dressing over the chickpea mixture. Toss until well coated.

4. Serve immediately or refrigerate for later. This salad can be enjoyed on its own or served over a bed of lettuce.

Turkey and Avocado Sandwich:

- Ingredients:
    1. 2 slices whole grain bread
    2. 2-3 slices turkey breast
    3. 1/4 avocado, sliced
    4. Handful of spinach leaves
    5. Mustard or mayonnaise (optional)
- Instructions:
    1. Toast the whole grain bread until golden brown.
    2. Spread mustard or mayonnaise (if using) on one slice of bread.
    3. Layer turkey breast, sliced avocado, and spinach leaves on top of the spread.

4. Place the second slice of bread on top to form a sandwich.

5. Slice in half diagonally and serve immediately, or wrap in foil for a portable lunch.

Vegetable Stir-Fry with Brown Rice:

- Ingredients:
    1. 1 cup cooked brown rice
    2. 1 cup mixed vegetables (such as bell peppers, broccoli, carrots, snap peas)
    3. 1 tablespoon olive oil
    4. 2 tablespoons low-sodium soy sauce
    5. 1 clove garlic, minced
    6. Optional: cooked chicken, tofu, or shrimp for added protein
- Instructions:

1. In a large skillet or wok, heat olive oil over medium-high heat.
2. Add minced garlic and cook for 1 minute, until fragrant.
3. Add mixed vegetables to the skillet and stir-fry for 5-7 minutes, or until vegetables are tender-crisp.
4. If using protein (such as chicken, tofu, or shrimp), add it to the skillet and cook until heated through.
5. Stir in cooked brown rice and soy sauce, tossing until well combined and heated through.
6. Serve hot as a flavorful and satisfying lunch option.

Tuna Salad Lettuce Wraps:

- Ingredients:

1. 1 can (5 oz) tuna, drained
2. 2 tablespoons Greek yogurt or mayonnaise
3. 1 tablespoon diced red onion
4. 1 tablespoon diced celery
5. 1 tablespoon chopped pickles
6. Salt and pepper to taste
7. Lettuce leaves for wrapping

- Instructions:
    1. In a bowl, mix together tuna, Greek yogurt or mayonnaise, diced red onion, diced celery, and chopped pickles.
    2. Season with salt and pepper to taste.
    3. Spoon the tuna salad onto lettuce leaves.
    4. Wrap the lettuce around the filling to form lettuce wraps.

5. Serve immediately as a light and refreshing lunch option.

Caprese Salad with Balsamic Glaze:

- Ingredients:
    1. 1 cup cherry tomatoes, halved
    2. 1 ball fresh mozzarella cheese, sliced
    3. Fresh basil leaves
    4. 2 tablespoons balsamic glaze
    5. Salt and pepper to taste
- Instructions:
    1. Arrange halved cherry tomatoes and sliced mozzarella cheese on a plate.
    2. Tuck fresh basil leaves in between the tomatoes and cheese slices.
    3. Drizzle balsamic glaze over the salad.

4. Season with salt and pepper to taste.
5. Serve immediately as a light and flavorful lunch option.

Vegetable Lentil Soup:

- Ingredients:
    1. 1 cup dried lentils
    2. 4 cups vegetable broth
    3. 1 onion, diced
    4. 2 carrots, diced
    5. 2 celery stalks, diced
    6. 2 cloves garlic, minced
    7. 1 teaspoon dried thyme
    8. Salt and pepper to taste
- Instructions:
    1. Rinse the lentils under cold water. In a large pot, combine lentils, vegetable broth, diced onion, diced carrots, diced celery, minced garlic, and dried thyme.

2. Bring to a boil, then reduce heat and simmer for 20-25 minutes, or until lentils and vegetables are tender.
3. Season with salt and pepper to taste.
4. Serve hot as a hearty and nutritious lunch option.

Turkey and Vegetable Stir-Fry:

- Ingredients:
    1. 1 tablespoon olive oil
    2. 1/2 lb turkey breast, sliced
    3. 2 cups mixed vegetables (such as bell peppers, broccoli, snap peas)
    4. 2 tablespoons low-sodium soy sauce
    5. 1 tablespoon honey or maple syrup
    6. 1 clove garlic, minced
    7. Cooked brown rice or quinoa for serving

- ○ Instructions:
    1. In a large skillet or wok, heat olive oil over medium-high heat.
    2. Add sliced turkey breast and cook until browned and cooked through, about 5-7 minutes.
    3. Add mixed vegetables and minced garlic to the skillet. Stir-fry for an additional 5 minutes, or until vegetables are tender-crisp.
    4. In a small bowl, whisk together soy sauce and honey or maple syrup. Pour over the turkey and vegetables in the skillet.
    5. Stir until everything is well coated and heated through.
    6. Serve hot over cooked brown rice or quinoa.

Salmon Salad Sandwich:

- Ingredients:
    1. 1 can (5 oz) salmon, drained
    2. 2 tablespoons Greek yogurt or mayonnaise
    3. 1 tablespoon chopped fresh dill
    4. 1 teaspoon lemon juice
    5. Salt and pepper to taste
    6. Lettuce leaves
    7. Whole grain bread slices
- Instructions:
    1. In a bowl, combine drained salmon, Greek yogurt or mayonnaise, chopped fresh dill, lemon juice, salt, and pepper.
    2. Mix well until everything is evenly combined.
    3. Place lettuce leaves on a slice of whole grain bread.
    4. Spoon the salmon salad onto the lettuce.

5. Top with another slice of bread to form a sandwich.

6. Slice in half diagonally and serve immediately, or wrap in foil for a portable lunch.

Chapter 13:DINNER RECIPES

Baked Lemon Herb Chicken:

- Ingredients:
    1. 2 boneless, skinless chicken breasts
    2. 2 tablespoons olive oil
    3. 2 cloves garlic, minced
    4. 1 teaspoon dried thyme
    5. 1 teaspoon dried rosemary
    6. 1 lemon, juiced and zested
    7. Salt and pepper to taste
- Instructions:
    1. Preheat oven to 400°F (200°C).
    2. In a small bowl, mix together olive oil, minced

garlic, dried thyme, dried rosemary, lemon juice, and lemon zest.

3. Place chicken breasts in a baking dish and season with salt and pepper.
4. Pour the lemon herb mixture over the chicken, ensuring it's evenly coated.
5. Bake for 20-25 minutes, or until chicken is cooked through and juices run clear.
6. Serve hot with your choice of side dishes, such as roasted vegetables or quinoa.

Vegetable Stir-Fry with Tofu:

- Ingredients:
  1. 1 block firm tofu, pressed and cubed
  2. 2 tablespoons soy sauce
  3. 1 tablespoon sesame oil

4. 1 tablespoon olive oil
5. 2 cups mixed vegetables (such as bell peppers, broccoli, carrots)
6. 2 cloves garlic, minced
7. Cooked brown rice for serving

- Instructions:
    1. In a bowl, toss cubed tofu with soy sauce and sesame oil. Let it marinate for 10-15 minutes.
    2. Heat olive oil in a large skillet or wok over medium-high heat.
    3. Add marinated tofu to the skillet and cook until golden brown on all sides, about 5-7 minutes. Remove tofu from the skillet and set aside.
    4. In the same skillet, add mixed vegetables and minced garlic. Stir-fry for

5-7 minutes, or until vegetables are tender-crisp.
        5. Return cooked tofu to the skillet and toss everything together until heated through.
        6. Serve hot over cooked brown rice.

Salmon with Roasted Vegetables:

- Ingredients:
    1. 2 salmon fillets
    2. 2 tablespoons olive oil
    3. 1 tablespoon lemon juice
    4. 1 teaspoon dried dill
    5. Salt and pepper to taste
    6. Assorted vegetables for roasting (such as potatoes, carrots, zucchini)
- Instructions:
    1. Preheat oven to 400°F (200°C).

2. In a small bowl, whisk together olive oil, lemon juice, dried dill, salt, and pepper.
3. Place salmon fillets on a baking sheet lined with parchment paper.
4. Brush the salmon fillets with the olive oil mixture, coating them evenly.
5. Arrange assorted vegetables around the salmon on the baking sheet.
6. Roast in the preheated oven for 15-20 minutes, or until salmon is cooked through and vegetables are tender.
7. Serve hot with a side of steamed rice or quinoa.

Turkey and Vegetable Skillet:

- Ingredients:

1. 1 lb ground turkey
2. 1 tablespoon olive oil
3. 1 onion, diced
4. 2 cloves garlic, minced
5. 2 cups mixed vegetables (such as bell peppers, mushrooms, spinach)
6. 1 can (14 oz) diced tomatoes
7. 1 teaspoon dried Italian seasoning
8. Salt and pepper to taste

- Instructions:
  1. Heat olive oil in a large skillet over medium heat.
  2. Add diced onion and minced garlic to the skillet. Cook until softened and fragrant, about 3-4 minutes.
  3. Add ground turkey to the skillet, breaking it up with a spatula. Cook until browned and cooked

through, about 5-7 minutes.

4. Stir in mixed vegetables, diced tomatoes, dried Italian seasoning, salt, and pepper.
5. Cook for an additional 5 minutes, or until vegetables are tender and flavors are well combined.
6. Serve hot as a hearty and satisfying dinner option.

Vegetarian Chili:

- Ingredients:
    1. 1 tablespoon olive oil
    2. 1 onion, diced
    3. 2 cloves garlic, minced
    4. 1 bell pepper, diced
    5. 1 zucchini, diced
    6. 1 can (14 oz) diced tomatoes
    7. 1 can (14 oz) kidney beans, drained and rinsed

8. 1 can (14 oz) black beans, drained and rinsed
9. 2 cups vegetable broth
10. 2 teaspoons chili powder
11. 1 teaspoon ground cumin
12. Salt and pepper to taste
- Instructions:
1. Heat olive oil in a large pot over medium heat.
2. Add diced onion and minced garlic to the pot. Cook until softened and fragrant, about 3-4 minutes.
3. Add diced bell pepper and zucchini to the pot. Cook for an additional 5 minutes, or until vegetables are softened.
4. Stir in diced tomatoes, kidney beans, black beans, vegetable broth, chili

powder, ground cumin, salt, and pepper.

5. Bring the chili to a simmer and cook for 20-25 minutes, stirring occasionally.
6. Serve hot with optional toppings such as shredded cheese, chopped cilantro, or a dollop of Greek yogurt.

Pasta Primavera:

- Ingredients:
  1. 8 oz whole wheat pasta
  2. 2 tablespoons olive oil
  3. 2 cloves garlic, minced
  4. 2 cups mixed vegetables (such as broccoli, bell peppers, cherry tomatoes)
  5. 1/4 cup grated Parmesan cheese
  6. Salt and pepper to taste

○ Instructions:
   1. Cook pasta according to package instructions until al dente. Drain and set aside.
   2. In a large skillet, heat olive oil over medium heat. Add minced garlic and cook until fragrant, about 1 minute.
   3. Add mixed vegetables to the skillet and sauté until tender, about 5-7 minutes.
   4. Toss cooked pasta with the sautéed vegetables in the skillet.
   5. Sprinkle grated Parmesan cheese over the pasta and vegetables. Season with salt and pepper to taste.
   6. Serve hot as a satisfying and flavorful dinner option.

Stuffed Bell Peppers:

- o Ingredients:
    1. 4 bell peppers, halved and seeds removed
    2. 1 cup cooked quinoa
    3. 1 can (15 oz) black beans, drained and rinsed
    4. 1 cup diced tomatoes
    5. 1 cup shredded cheddar cheese
    6. 1 teaspoon chili powder
    7. Salt and pepper to taste
- o Instructions:
    1. Preheat oven to 375°F (190°C).
    2. In a large bowl, mix together cooked quinoa, black beans, diced tomatoes, shredded cheddar cheese, chili powder, salt, and pepper.
    3. Stuff each bell pepper half with the quinoa mixture.

4. Place stuffed bell peppers in a baking dish and cover with aluminum foil.
5. Bake in the preheated oven for 25-30 minutes, or until peppers are tender and filling is heated through.
6. Serve hot as a hearty and nutritious dinner option.

Teriyaki Salmon with Stir-Fried Vegetables:

- Ingredients:
    1. 2 salmon fillets
    2. 1/4 cup teriyaki sauce
    3. 1 tablespoon olive oil
    4. 2 cups mixed vegetables (such as snap peas, carrots, bell peppers)
    5. Cooked brown rice for serving
- Instructions:

1. Marinate salmon fillets in teriyaki sauce for 20-30 minutes.
2. Heat olive oil in a large skillet over medium-high heat.
3. Add marinated salmon fillets to the skillet and cook for 3-4 minutes per side, or until salmon is cooked through and flakes easily with a fork.
4. Remove cooked salmon from the skillet and set aside.
5. In the same skillet, add mixed vegetables and stir-fry until tender-crisp, about 5-7 minutes.
6. Serve cooked salmon and stir-fried vegetables over cooked brown rice.

Vegetable Curry with Chickpeas:

- Ingredients:
    1. 1 tablespoon olive oil
    2. 1 onion, diced
    3. 2 cloves garlic, minced
    4. 2 teaspoons curry powder
    5. 1 teaspoon ground cumin
    6. 1 can (14 oz) diced tomatoes
    7. 1 can (14 oz) coconut milk
    8. 1 can (14 oz) chickpeas, drained and rinsed
    9. 2 cups mixed vegetables (such as cauliflower, bell peppers, peas)
    10. Cooked rice or naan bread for serving
- Instructions:
    1. Heat olive oil in a large pot over medium heat.
    2. Add diced onion and minced garlic to the pot. Cook until softened and

fragrant, about 3-4 minutes.

3. Stir in curry powder and ground cumin, and cook for an additional 1-2 minutes.
4. Add diced tomatoes, coconut milk, chickpeas, and mixed vegetables to the pot. Bring to a simmer and cook for 15-20 minutes, stirring occasionally.
5. Serve hot over cooked rice or with naan bread for dipping.

Grilled Vegetable Quesadillas:

- Ingredients:
  1. 4 large whole wheat tortillas
  2. 1 cup shredded cheese (such as cheddar or Monterey Jack)

3. 2 cups mixed grilled vegetables (such as zucchini, bell peppers, onions)
4. Olive oil for brushing
5. Guacamole and salsa for serving (optional)

- Instructions:
    1. Preheat a grill or grill pan over medium-high heat.
    2. Brush both sides of each tortilla lightly with olive oil.
    3. Place tortillas on the grill and cook for 1-2 minutes on each side, until lightly charred and grill marks appear.
    4. Remove tortillas from the grill and lay them flat on a clean surface.
    5. Sprinkle shredded cheese evenly over half of each

tortilla. Top with grilled vegetables.

6. Fold the tortillas in half to cover the filling, creating quesadillas.

7. Return quesadillas to the grill and cook for an additional 2-3 minutes on each side, until cheese is melted and filling is heated through.

8. Slice quesadillas into wedges and serve hot with guacamole and salsa on the side, if desired.

Chapter 14:APPETIZERS AND SNACKS RECIPES

Hummus with Crudites:

- Ingredients:
    1. 1 can (15 oz) chickpeas, drained and rinsed

2. 2 tablespoons tahini
   3. 2 tablespoons lemon juice
   4. 1 clove garlic, minced
   5. 2 tablespoons olive oil
   6. Salt and pepper to taste
   7. Assorted raw vegetables (such as carrot sticks, cucumber slices, bell pepper strips)
- Instructions:
   1. In a food processor, combine chickpeas, tahini, lemon juice, minced garlic, olive oil, salt, and pepper.
   2. Blend until smooth and creamy, adding a little water if needed to achieve desired consistency.
   3. Transfer hummus to a serving bowl and garnish with a drizzle of olive oil and a sprinkle of paprika, if desired.

4. Serve with assorted raw vegetables for dipping.

Greek Yogurt Dip with Pita Chips:

- Ingredients:
    1. 1 cup Greek yogurt
    2. 1 tablespoon lemon juice
    3. 1 teaspoon dried dill
    4. 1/2 teaspoon garlic powder
    5. Salt and pepper to taste
    6. Whole wheat pita bread, cut into wedges
- Instructions:
    1. In a bowl, mix together Greek yogurt, lemon juice, dried dill, garlic powder, salt, and pepper.
    2. Adjust seasoning to taste.
    3. Serve the yogurt dip with whole wheat pita wedges for dipping.

Avocado Toast with Cherry Tomatoes:

- Ingredients:

1. 2 slices whole grain bread
2. 1 ripe avocado
3. 1/2 cup cherry tomatoes, halved
4. Salt and pepper to taste
5. Optional: red pepper flakes, chopped cilantro

- Instructions:
    1. Toast the whole grain bread until golden brown.
    2. Mash the ripe avocado and spread it evenly onto the toasted bread slices.
    3. Top avocado toast with halved cherry tomatoes.
    4. Season with salt and pepper to taste.
    5. Sprinkle with optional red pepper flakes and chopped cilantro for added flavor.
    6. Serve immediately as a delicious and nutritious snack.

Trail Mix with Nuts and Dried Fruit:

- Ingredients:
    1. 1 cup mixed nuts (such as almonds, walnuts, cashews)
    2. 1/2 cup dried fruit (such as raisins, cranberries, apricots)
    3. 1/4 cup dark chocolate chips (optional)
    4. 1/4 teaspoon cinnamon (optional)
- Instructions:
    1. In a bowl, combine mixed nuts, dried fruit, dark chocolate chips, and cinnamon (if using).
    2. Toss everything together until well mixed.
    3. Transfer trail mix to an airtight container for storage.

4. Enjoy a handful of trail mix as a quick and satisfying snack.

Caprese Skewers:

- Ingredients:
    1. Cherry tomatoes
    2. Fresh mozzarella cheese, cut into cubes
    3. Fresh basil leaves
    4. Balsamic glaze for drizzling
    5. Toothpicks or small skewers
- Instructions:
    1. Thread one cherry tomato, one cube of fresh mozzarella cheese, and one fresh basil leaf onto each toothpick or skewer.
    2. Arrange caprese skewers on a serving platter.
    3. Drizzle balsamic glaze over the skewers.

4. Serve immediately as a light and flavorful appetizer.

Chapter 15:HEALTHY RECIPES

Quinoa Salad with Chicken and Avocado:
- Ingredients:
    1. 1 cup quinoa, rinsed
    2. 2 cups water or chicken broth
    3. 1 boneless, skinless chicken breast
    4. 1 avocado, diced
    5. 1 cup cherry tomatoes, halved
    6. 1/4 cup chopped fresh cilantro
    7. 2 tablespoons olive oil
    8. 1 tablespoon lime juice
    9. Salt and pepper to taste
- Instructions:

1. In a medium saucepan, bring water or chicken broth to a boil. Add quinoa, reduce heat to low, cover, and simmer for 15-20 minutes, or until quinoa is cooked and water is absorbed.

2. Meanwhile, season chicken breast with salt and pepper. Grill or cook in a skillet over medium heat until cooked through, about 6-8 minutes per side. Let it rest for a few minutes, then slice thinly.

3. In a large bowl, combine cooked quinoa, sliced chicken breast, diced avocado, cherry tomatoes, and chopped cilantro.

4. In a small bowl, whisk together olive oil and lime juice to make the dressing.

Pour over the salad and toss until well combined.

5. Season with additional salt and pepper to taste, if needed.

6. Serve chilled or at room temperature as a nutritious and satisfying meal.

Salmon and Vegetable Foil Packets:

- Ingredients:
    1. 2 salmon fillets
    2. 2 cups mixed vegetables (such as broccoli, bell peppers, carrots)
    3. 2 tablespoons olive oil
    4. 2 cloves garlic, minced
    5. 1 tablespoon lemon juice
    6. Salt and pepper to taste
- Instructions:
    1. Preheat oven to 400°F (200°C).

2. Cut two large pieces of aluminum foil. Place one salmon fillet in the center of each piece of foil.

3. In a bowl, toss mixed vegetables with olive oil, minced garlic, lemon juice, salt, and pepper.

4. Divide the vegetable mixture evenly between the two foil packets, arranging them around the salmon fillets.

5. Fold the edges of the foil over the salmon and vegetables to create sealed packets.

6. Place foil packets on a baking sheet and bake in the preheated oven for 15-20 minutes, or until salmon is cooked through and vegetables are tender.

7. Carefully open the foil packets and serve hot.

Turkey and Quinoa Stuffed Bell Peppers:

- Ingredients:
    1. 4 large bell peppers, tops removed and seeds removed
    2. 1 cup quinoa, rinsed
    3. 2 cups water or vegetable broth
    4. 1 lb lean ground turkey
    5. 1 onion, diced
    6. 2 cloves garlic, minced
    7. 1 can (14 oz) diced tomatoes
    8. 1 teaspoon dried oregano
    9. 1 teaspoon dried basil
    10. Salt and pepper to taste
- Instructions:
    1. Preheat oven to 375°F (190°C).
    2. In a medium saucepan, bring water or vegetable

broth to a boil. Add quinoa, reduce heat to low, cover, and simmer for 15-20 minutes, or until quinoa is cooked and water is absorbed.

3. In a large skillet, cook ground turkey over medium heat until browned and cooked through, breaking it up with a spatula. Drain any excess fat.

4. Add diced onion and minced garlic to the skillet with the turkey. Cook until softened, about 3-4 minutes.

5. Stir in diced tomatoes, cooked quinoa, dried oregano, dried basil, salt, and pepper. Cook for an additional 5 minutes, until heated through.

6. Spoon the turkey and quinoa mixture evenly into the hollowed-out bell peppers.
7. Place stuffed bell peppers in a baking dish and cover with aluminum foil.
8. Bake in the preheated oven for 25-30 minutes, or until peppers are tender.
9. Serve hot as a nutritious and filling meal.

Vegetable and Lentil Soup:

- Ingredients:
    1. 1 tablespoon olive oil
    2. 1 onion, diced
    3. 2 carrots, diced
    4. 2 celery stalks, diced
    5. 2 cloves garlic, minced
    6. 1 cup dried green lentils, rinsed
    7. 6 cups vegetable broth

8. 1 can (14 oz) diced tomatoes
9. 2 cups chopped spinach or kale
10. 1 teaspoon dried thyme
11. Salt and pepper to taste

- Instructions:
  1. In a large pot, heat olive oil over medium heat.
  2. Add diced onion, carrots, and celery to the pot. Cook until softened, about 5-7 minutes.
  3. Add minced garlic and cook for an additional minute, until fragrant.
  4. Stir in dried lentils, vegetable broth, diced tomatoes (with their juices), chopped spinach or kale, dried thyme, salt, and pepper.
  5. Bring the soup to a boil, then reduce heat to low

and simmer for 25-30 minutes, or until lentils are tender.

6. Adjust seasoning to taste before serving.
7. Serve hot as a comforting and nutritious meal.

Mediterranean Chicken Skewers with Tzatziki Sauce:

- Ingredients:
    1. 2 boneless, skinless chicken breasts, cut into chunks
    2. 1 tablespoon olive oil
    3. 1 tablespoon lemon juice
    4. 1 teaspoon dried oregano
    5. Salt and pepper to taste
    6. Cherry tomatoes, halved
    7. Red onion, cut into chunks
    8. Wooden skewers, soaked in water for 30 minutes
    9. Tzatziki sauce for serving
- Instructions:

1. In a bowl, combine chicken chunks with olive oil, lemon juice, dried oregano, salt, and pepper. Let it marinate for at least 30 minutes.
2. Preheat grill or grill pan over medium-high heat.
3. Thread marinated chicken chunks onto soaked wooden skewers, alternating with cherry tomatoes and red onion chunks.
4. Grill skewers for 6-8 minutes per side, or until chicken is cooked through and juices run clear.
5. Serve hot skewers with tzatziki sauce for dipping.

Vegetable Lentil Soup:

- o Ingredients:
    1. 1 cup dried green lentils, rinsed
    2. 6 cups vegetable broth
    3. 1 onion, diced
    4. 2 carrots, diced
    5. 2 celery stalks, diced
    6. 2 cloves garlic, minced
    7. 1 can (14 oz) diced tomatoes
    8. 2 cups chopped spinach or kale
    9. 1 teaspoon dried thyme
    10. Salt and pepper to taste
- o Instructions:
    1. In a large pot, combine dried lentils, vegetable broth, diced onion, diced carrots, diced celery, minced garlic, diced

tomatoes (with their juices), chopped spinach or kale, dried thyme, salt, and pepper.
2. Bring the soup to a boil over medium-high heat.
3. Reduce heat to low, cover, and simmer for 25-30 minutes, or until lentils and vegetables are tender.
4. Adjust seasoning to taste before serving.
5. Serve hot as a comforting and nutritious meal.

Chicken and Vegetable Soup:

- Ingredients:
    1. 1 tablespoon olive oil
    2. 1 onion, diced
    3. 2 carrots, diced
    4. 2 celery stalks, diced
    5. 2 cloves garlic, minced
    6. 6 cups chicken broth

7. 2 boneless, skinless chicken breasts, cooked and shredded
8. 1 can (14 oz) diced tomatoes
9. 1 cup chopped spinach or kale
10. 1 teaspoon dried thyme
11. Salt and pepper to taste

- Instructions:
    1. In a large pot, heat olive oil over medium heat.
    2. Add diced onion, carrots, and celery to the pot. Cook until softened, about 5-7 minutes.
    3. Add minced garlic and cook for an additional minute, until fragrant.
    4. Pour in chicken broth and bring to a simmer.
    5. Stir in shredded chicken, diced tomatoes (with their juices), chopped spinach

or kale, dried thyme, salt, and pepper.

6. Simmer for 15-20 minutes, allowing flavors to meld together.
7. Adjust seasoning to taste before serving.
8. Serve hot as a hearty and nourishing meal.

Tomato Basil Soup:

- Ingredients:
    1. 2 tablespoons olive oil
    2. 1 onion, diced
    3. 2 cloves garlic, minced
    4. 2 cans (14 oz each) diced tomatoes
    5. 2 cups vegetable broth
    6. 1/2 cup fresh basil leaves, chopped
    7. Salt and pepper to taste
    8. Optional: 1/4 cup heavy cream or coconut milk
- Instructions:

1. In a large pot, heat olive oil over medium heat.
2. Add diced onion to the pot and cook until softened, about 5 minutes.
3. Add minced garlic and cook for an additional minute, until fragrant.
4. Pour in diced tomatoes (with their juices) and vegetable broth. Bring to a simmer.
5. Simmer for 15-20 minutes to allow flavors to develop.
6. Stir in chopped basil leaves and season with salt and pepper to taste.
7. If using, stir in heavy cream or coconut milk for added richness.
8. Use an immersion blender or transfer soup to a blender to puree until smooth.

9. Serve hot garnished with additional fresh basil leaves, if desired.

Minestrone Soup:

- Ingredients:
    1. 2 tablespoons olive oil
    2. 1 onion, diced
    3. 2 carrots, diced
    4. 2 celery stalks, diced
    5. 2 cloves garlic, minced
    6. 1 can (14 oz) diced tomatoes
    7. 6 cups vegetable broth
    8. 1 can (15 oz) kidney beans, drained and rinsed
    9. 1 cup small pasta (such as ditalini or elbow)
    10. 2 cups chopped spinach or kale
    11. 1 teaspoon dried oregano
    12. 1 teaspoon dried basil
    13. Salt and pepper to taste
- Instructions:

1. In a large pot, heat olive oil over medium heat.
2. Add diced onion, carrots, and celery to the pot. Cook until softened, about 5-7 minutes.
3. Add minced garlic and cook for an additional minute, until fragrant.
4. Stir in diced tomatoes (with their juices), vegetable broth, kidney beans, pasta, dried oregano, and dried basil.
5. Bring to a boil, then reduce heat to low and simmer for 10-15 minutes, or until pasta is cooked and vegetables are tender.
6. Stir in chopped spinach or kale and cook for an additional 2-3 minutes, until wilted.

7. Season with salt and pepper to taste before serving.
8. Serve hot as a satisfying and flavorful meal.

Beef and Barley Stew:

- Ingredients:
    1. 1 tablespoon olive oil
    2. 1 lb stew beef, cut into bite-sized pieces
    3. 1 onion, diced
    4. 2 carrots, diced
    5. 2 celery stalks, diced
    6. 2 cloves garlic, minced
    7. 6 cups beef broth
    8. 1 cup pearl barley
    9. 2 bay leaves
    10. Salt and pepper to taste
- Instructions:
    1. In a large pot, heat olive oil over medium heat.
    2. Add stew beef to the pot and cook until browned on

all sides, about 5-7 minutes.

3. Add diced onion, carrots, and celery to the pot. Cook until softened, about 5 minutes.

4. Add minced garlic and cook for an additional minute, until fragrant.

5. Pour in beef broth and stir in pearl barley and bay leaves.

6. Bring to a boil, then reduce heat to low and simmer for 45-60 minutes, or until beef is tender and barley is cooked.

7. Remove bay leaves and season with salt and pepper to taste before serving.

8. Serve hot as a hearty and comforting stew.

Vegetable Stir-Fry:

- Ingredients:
    1. Assorted vegetables (such as bell peppers, broccoli, carrots, snap peas, mushrooms)
    2. 2 tablespoons soy sauce
    3. 1 tablespoon sesame oil
    4. 1 tablespoon olive oil
    5. 2 cloves garlic, minced
    6. 1 tablespoon grated ginger
    7. Cooked rice or noodles for serving
- Instructions:
    1. Heat olive oil in a large skillet or wok over medium-high heat.
    2. Add minced garlic and grated ginger to the skillet

and cook for 1-2 minutes until fragrant.

3. Add assorted vegetables to the skillet and stir-fry for 5-7 minutes until tender-crisp.
4. In a small bowl, whisk together soy sauce and sesame oil. Pour the sauce over the vegetables and toss to coat evenly.
5. Serve the vegetable stir-fry over cooked rice or noodles.

Mushroom Risotto:

- Ingredients:
    1. 1 cup Arborio rice
    2. 4 cups vegetable broth
    3. 2 tablespoons olive oil
    4. 1 onion, diced
    5. 2 cloves garlic, minced
    6. 8 oz mushrooms, sliced

7. 1/2 cup grated Parmesan cheese

8. Salt and pepper to taste

- Instructions:

  1. In a medium saucepan, heat vegetable broth over medium heat until simmering.

  2. In a separate large skillet, heat olive oil over medium heat. Add diced onion and minced garlic, and cook until softened.

  3. Add Arborio rice to the skillet and cook for 1-2 minutes until lightly toasted.

  4. Gradually add simmering vegetable broth to the skillet, one ladleful at a time, stirring constantly until the liquid is absorbed before adding more.

5. Continue this process until the rice is creamy and tender, about 20-25 minutes.
6. Stir in sliced mushrooms and cook for an additional 5 minutes until mushrooms are cooked through.
7. Remove from heat and stir in grated Parmesan cheese. Season with salt and pepper to taste.
8. Serve hot as a comforting and flavorful vegetarian main dish.

Vegetarian Chili:

- Ingredients:
    1. 1 tablespoon olive oil
    2. 1 onion, diced
    3. 2 cloves garlic, minced
    4. 1 bell pepper, diced
    5. 1 zucchini, diced

6. 1 can (14 oz) diced tomatoes
7. 1 can (14 oz) black beans, drained and rinsed
8. 1 can (14 oz) kidney beans, drained and rinsed
9. 1 cup vegetable broth
10. 2 tablespoons chili powder
11. 1 teaspoon cumin
12. Salt and pepper to taste

- Instructions:
    1. Heat olive oil in a large pot over medium heat. Add diced onion and minced garlic, and cook until softened.
    2. Add diced bell pepper and zucchini to the pot, and cook for 5 minutes until slightly softened.
    3. Stir in diced tomatoes, black beans, kidney beans, vegetable broth, chili

powder, cumin, salt, and pepper.

4. Bring the chili to a simmer and cook for 20-25 minutes until flavors are blended and vegetables are tender.
5. Adjust seasoning to taste before serving.
6. Serve hot with your favorite toppings such as shredded cheese, sour cream, or chopped cilantro.

Caprese Stuffed Portobello Mushrooms:

- Ingredients:
    1. 4 large portobello mushrooms
    2. 2 tablespoons olive oil
    3. 2 cloves garlic, minced
    4. 2 large tomatoes, sliced
    5. 8 oz fresh mozzarella cheese, sliced

6. Fresh basil leaves
7. Balsamic glaze for drizzling
8. Salt and pepper to taste

- Instructions:
    1. Preheat oven to 400°F (200°C). Remove stems from portobello mushrooms and gently scrape out the gills.
    2. In a small bowl, mix together olive oil and minced garlic. Brush the inside of each mushroom cap with the garlic-infused oil.
    3. Place mushroom caps on a baking sheet lined with parchment paper. Season with salt and pepper.
    4. Layer sliced tomatoes, fresh mozzarella slices, and fresh basil leaves

inside each mushroom cap.
5. Bake in the preheated oven for 15-20 minutes, or until cheese is melted and mushrooms are tender.
6. Drizzle with balsamic glaze before serving.

Vegetable Paella:

- Ingredients:
    1. 2 tablespoons olive oil
    2. 1 onion, diced
    3. 2 cloves garlic, minced
    4. 1 bell pepper, diced
    5. 1 zucchini, diced
    6. 1 cup Arborio rice
    7. 2 cups vegetable broth
    8. 1 teaspoon smoked paprika
    9. 1/2 teaspoon saffron threads (optional)
    10. 1 cup frozen peas
    11. Salt and pepper to taste

- Instructions:
  1. Heat olive oil in a large skillet or paella pan over medium heat. Add diced onion and minced garlic, and cook until softened.
  2. Add diced bell pepper and zucchini to the skillet, and cook for 5 minutes until slightly softened.
  3. Stir in Arborio rice, smoked paprika, and saffron threads (if using). Cook for 1-2 minutes until rice is coated with oil.
  4. Pour vegetable broth into the skillet and bring to a simmer. Reduce heat to low, cover, and cook for 15-20 minutes until rice is tender and liquid is absorbed.
  5. Stir in frozen peas and cook for an additional 2-3

minutes until peas are heated through.

6. Season with salt and pepper to taste before serving.
7. Serve hot as a flavorful and satisfying vegetarian main dish.

Chapter 18:POULTRY AND SEAFOOD RECIPES

Lemon Garlic Roasted Chicken:

- o Ingredients:
    1. 4 bone-in, skin-on chicken thighs
    2. 2 tablespoons olive oil
    3. 2 cloves garlic, minced
    4. 1 lemon, juiced and zest
    5. 1 teaspoon dried thyme
    6. Salt and pepper to taste
- o Instructions:
    1. Preheat oven to 400°F (200°C).

2. In a small bowl, whisk together olive oil, minced garlic, lemon juice, lemon zest, dried thyme, salt, and pepper.

3. Place chicken thighs in a baking dish and pour the lemon garlic mixture over them, ensuring they are evenly coated.

4. Roast in the preheated oven for 30-35 minutes, or until the chicken is cooked through and the skin is crispy.

5. Serve hot with your favorite side dishes.

Baked Salmon with Herbs:

- Ingredients:
    1. 4 salmon fillets
    2. 2 tablespoons olive oil
    3. 2 tablespoons chopped fresh dill

    4. 2 tablespoons chopped fresh parsley
    5. 2 cloves garlic, minced
    6. 1 lemon, thinly sliced
    7. Salt and pepper to taste
- Instructions:
  1. Preheat oven to 400°F (200°C).
  2. Place salmon fillets on a baking sheet lined with parchment paper.
  3. In a small bowl, mix together olive oil, chopped fresh dill, chopped fresh parsley, minced garlic, salt, and pepper.
  4. Brush the herb mixture over the salmon fillets, then top each fillet with lemon slices.
  5. Bake in the preheated oven for 12-15 minutes, or until the salmon is cooked

through and flakes easily with a fork.

6. Serve hot with steamed vegetables or a salad.

Grilled Chicken Skewers:

- Ingredients:
    1. 1 lb chicken breast, cut into cubes
    2. 2 tablespoons olive oil
    3. 1 tablespoon lemon juice
    4. 1 teaspoon dried oregano
    5. Salt and pepper to taste
    6. Wooden skewers, soaked in water for 30 minutes
- Instructions:
    1. In a bowl, combine chicken cubes with olive oil, lemon juice, dried oregano, salt, and pepper. Let it marinate for at least 30 minutes.
    2. Preheat grill or grill pan over medium-high heat.

3. Thread marinated chicken cubes onto soaked wooden skewers.
4. Grill skewers for 6-8 minutes per side, or until chicken is cooked through and juices run clear.
5. Serve hot with rice and grilled vegetables.

Shrimp Stir-Fry:

- Ingredients:
    1. 1 lb shrimp, peeled and deveined
    2. 2 tablespoons soy sauce
    3. 1 tablespoon sesame oil
    4. 1 tablespoon olive oil
    5. 2 cloves garlic, minced
    6. 1 teaspoon grated ginger
    7. Assorted vegetables (such as bell peppers, broccoli, carrots, snap peas)
    8. Cooked rice for serving
- Instructions:

1. In a bowl, toss shrimp with soy sauce and sesame oil. Let it marinate for 15-20 minutes.
2. Heat olive oil in a large skillet or wok over medium-high heat.
3. Add minced garlic and grated ginger to the skillet and cook for 1-2 minutes until fragrant.
4. Add assorted vegetables to the skillet and stir-fry for 5-7 minutes until tender-crisp.
5. Push the vegetables to one side of the skillet and add the marinated shrimp. Cook for 2-3 minutes per side until pink and cooked through.
6. Serve the shrimp stir-fry over cooked rice.

Lemon Herb Baked Cod:

- Ingredients:
    1. 4 cod fillets
    2. 2 tablespoons olive oil
    3. 2 tablespoons chopped fresh parsley
    4. 2 tablespoons chopped fresh dill
    5. 2 cloves garlic, minced
    6. 1 lemon, juiced and zest
    7. Salt and pepper to taste
- Instructions:
    1. Preheat oven to 400°F (200°C).
    2. Place cod fillets on a baking sheet lined with parchment paper.
    3. In a small bowl, mix together olive oil, chopped fresh parsley, chopped fresh dill, minced garlic, lemon juice, lemon zest, salt, and pepper.

4. Brush the herb mixture over the cod fillets.
5. Bake in the preheated oven for 12-15 minutes, or until the cod is cooked through and flakes easily with a fork.
6. Serve hot with roasted vegetables or a side salad.

Chapter 19: RED MEAT DISHES RECIPES

Beef Stir-Fry:

- Ingredients:
    1. 1 lb beef steak (such as sirloin or flank), thinly sliced
    2. 2 tablespoons soy sauce
    3. 1 tablespoon sesame oil
    4. 1 tablespoon olive oil
    5. 2 cloves garlic, minced
    6. 1 teaspoon grated ginger

7. Assorted vegetables (such as bell peppers, broccoli, carrots, snap peas)
8. Cooked rice or noodles for serving

- Instructions:
    1. In a bowl, toss beef slices with soy sauce and sesame oil. Let it marinate for 15-20 minutes.
    2. Heat olive oil in a large skillet or wok over medium-high heat.
    3. Add minced garlic and grated ginger to the skillet and cook for 1-2 minutes until fragrant.
    4. Add assorted vegetables to the skillet and stir-fry for 5-7 minutes until tender-crisp.
    5. Push the vegetables to one side of the skillet and add the marinated beef slices.

Cook for 2-3 minutes per side until browned and cooked through.

6. Serve the beef stir-fry over cooked rice or noodles.

Beef and Vegetable Skewers:

- Ingredients:
  1. 1 lb beef sirloin, cut into cubes
  2. Assorted vegetables (such as bell peppers, onions, cherry tomatoes, mushrooms)
  3. 2 tablespoons olive oil
  4. 2 tablespoons balsamic vinegar
  5. 2 cloves garlic, minced
  6. Salt and pepper to taste
  7. Wooden skewers, soaked in water for 30 minutes
- Instructions:
  1. In a bowl, mix together olive oil, balsamic vinegar,

minced garlic, salt, and pepper.

2. Thread beef cubes and assorted vegetables onto soaked wooden skewers.
3. Brush the skewers with the marinade mixture.
4. Preheat grill or grill pan over medium-high heat.
5. Grill skewers for 8-10 minutes, turning occasionally, until beef is cooked to desired doneness and vegetables are tender.
6. Serve hot with a side of rice or salad.

Beef and Broccoli Stir-Fry:

- Ingredients:
    1. 1 lb beef sirloin, thinly sliced
    2. 2 tablespoons soy sauce
    3. 1 tablespoon olive oil

4. 2 cloves garlic, minced
5. 1 teaspoon grated ginger
6. 1 head broccoli, cut into florets
7. Cooked rice for serving

o Instructions:

1. In a bowl, toss beef slices with soy sauce. Let it marinate for 15-20 minutes.
2. Heat olive oil in a large skillet or wok over medium-high heat.
3. Add minced garlic and grated ginger to the skillet and cook for 1-2 minutes until fragrant.
4. Add broccoli florets to the skillet and stir-fry for 5-7 minutes until tender-crisp.
5. Push the broccoli to one side of the skillet and add the marinated beef slices. Cook for 2-3 minutes per

side until browned and cooked through.

6. Serve the beef and broccoli stir-fry over cooked rice.

Beef Chili:

- Ingredients:
    1. 1 lb ground beef
    2. 1 onion, diced
    3. 2 cloves garlic, minced
    4. 1 bell pepper, diced
    5. 1 can (14 oz) diced tomatoes
    6. 1 can (14 oz) kidney beans, drained and rinsed
    7. 1 cup beef broth
    8. 2 tablespoons chili powder
    9. 1 teaspoon cumin
    10. Salt and pepper to taste
- Instructions:
    1. In a large pot, cook ground beef over medium heat until browned.

2. Add diced onion, minced garlic, and diced bell pepper to the pot, and cook until softened.
3. Stir in diced tomatoes, kidney beans, beef broth, chili powder, cumin, salt, and pepper.
4. Bring the chili to a simmer and cook for 20-25 minutes until flavors are blended and vegetables are tender.
5. Adjust seasoning to taste before serving.
6. Serve hot with your favorite toppings such as shredded cheese, sour cream, or chopped cilantro.

Beef and Mushroom Skillet:

- Ingredients:

1. 1 lb beef sirloin, thinly sliced
2. 2 tablespoons olive oil
3. 2 cloves garlic, minced
4. 8 oz mushrooms, sliced
5. 1 onion, sliced
6. 1 bell pepper, sliced
7. 1 teaspoon dried thyme
8. Salt and pepper to taste

- Instructions:
    1. Heat olive oil in a large skillet over medium-high heat.
    2. Add minced garlic to the skillet and cook for 1-2 minutes until fragrant.
    3. Add sliced mushrooms, onion, and bell pepper to the skillet, and cook for 5-7 minutes until softened.
    4. Push the vegetables to one side of the skillet and add the thinly sliced beef. Cook for 2-3 minutes per side

until browned and cooked through.

5. Sprinkle dried thyme over the beef and vegetables. Season with salt and pepper to taste.
6. Serve hot as a hearty and satisfying meal.

Chapter 20: DESSERT RECIPES

Banana Oat Cookies:

- Ingredients:
    1. 2 ripe bananas, mashed
    2. 1 cup rolled oats
    3. 1/4 cup raisins or chocolate chips (optional)
    4. 1/4 teaspoon cinnamon (optional)
- Instructions:
    1. Preheat oven to 350°F (175°C). Line a baking

sheet with parchment paper.

2. In a bowl, combine mashed bananas, rolled oats, raisins or chocolate chips (if using), and cinnamon (if using). Mix until well combined.
3. Drop spoonfuls of the mixture onto the prepared baking sheet, spacing them apart.
4. Flatten each cookie with the back of a spoon.
5. Bake in the preheated oven for 12-15 minutes, or until golden brown.
6. Allow cookies to cool on the baking sheet for a few minutes before transferring to a wire rack to cool completely.

Frozen Banana Bites:

- Ingredients:
    1. 2 ripe bananas
    2. 1/4 cup peanut butter or almond butter
    3. 1/4 cup dark chocolate chips
    4. 1 tablespoon coconut oil
    5. Crushed nuts or shredded coconut for coating (optional)
- Instructions:
    1. Peel the bananas and cut them into thick slices.
    2. Spread peanut butter or almond butter on half of the banana slices, then top with the remaining slices to make sandwiches.
    3. Place the banana sandwiches on a baking sheet lined with parchment paper and

freeze for 1-2 hours until firm.

4. In a microwave-safe bowl, melt dark chocolate chips and coconut oil in 30-second intervals, stirring until smooth.

5. Dip each frozen banana sandwich into the melted chocolate, allowing any excess to drip off.

6. Roll the chocolate-coated bananas in crushed nuts or shredded coconut if desired.

7. Place the banana bites back on the parchment-lined baking sheet and freeze for an additional 30 minutes until the chocolate sets.

8. Serve cold as a delicious frozen treat.

Apple Crisp:

- Ingredients:
    1. 4 cups sliced apples
    2. 1 tablespoon lemon juice
    3. 1/2 cup rolled oats
    4. 1/4 cup all-purpose flour
    5. 1/4 cup brown sugar
    6. 1/4 teaspoon cinnamon
    7. 2 tablespoons butter, melted
- Instructions:
    1. Preheat oven to 350°F (175°C). Grease a baking dish with butter or cooking spray.
    2. In a bowl, toss sliced apples with lemon juice and spread them evenly in the prepared baking dish.
    3. In a separate bowl, combine rolled oats, all-purpose flour, brown sugar, cinnamon, and

melted butter. Mix until crumbly.

4. Sprinkle the oat mixture over the sliced apples in the baking dish.
5. Bake in the preheated oven for 30-35 minutes, or until the topping is golden brown and the apples are tender.
6. Allow the apple crisp to cool slightly before serving.
7. Serve warm with a scoop of vanilla ice cream or a dollop of whipped cream.

Greek Yogurt Parfait:

- Ingredients:
  1. 1 cup Greek yogurt
  2. 1/2 cup granola
  3. 1/2 cup mixed berries (such as strawberries, blueberries, raspberries)

4. 1 tablespoon honey (optional)
   ○ Instructions:
      1. In a glass or bowl, layer Greek yogurt, granola, and mixed berries.
      2. Repeat the layers until the glass or bowl is filled.
      3. Drizzle honey over the top if desired.
      4. Serve immediately as a nutritious and refreshing dessert or snack.

Chocolate Avocado Mousse:

   ○ Ingredients:
      1. 2 ripe avocados
      2. 1/4 cup cocoa powder
      3. 1/4 cup maple syrup or honey
      4. 1 teaspoon vanilla extract
      5. Pinch of salt
   ○ Instructions:

1. Scoop the flesh of the avocados into a blender or food processor.
2. Add cocoa powder, maple syrup or honey, vanilla extract, and a pinch of salt.
3. Blend until smooth and creamy, scraping down the sides as needed.
4. Transfer the chocolate avocado mousse to serving bowls or glasses.
5. Chill in the refrigerator for at least 30 minutes before serving.
6. Serve cold, optionally topped with whipped cream or fresh berries.

Chapter 21:28DAY MEAL PLAN

Day 1:

- Breakfast: Vegetable Omelette (eggs, bell peppers, spinach, onions) served with whole grain toast.
- Lunch: Quinoa Salad with Chickpeas, Cherry Tomatoes, Cucumber, and Lemon-Tahini Dressing.
- Dinner: Baked Salmon with Herbs (salmon fillets marinated with olive oil, dill, parsley, garlic, lemon) served with roasted sweet potatoes and steamed broccoli.

Day 2:

- Breakfast: Greek Yogurt Parfait (Greek yogurt layered with granola and mixed berries).
- Lunch: Lentil Soup with Spinach and Carrots served with a side of whole grain bread.

- Dinner: Vegetable Stir-Fry (assorted vegetables stir-fried with tofu or chicken) served with brown rice.

Day 3:

- Breakfast: Banana Oatmeal (oatmeal topped with sliced bananas, chopped nuts, and a drizzle of honey).
- Lunch: Caprese Stuffed Portobello Mushrooms served with a side salad.
- Dinner: Beef and Broccoli Stir-Fry (thinly sliced beef stir-fried with broccoli and garlic) served with quinoa.

Day 4:

- Breakfast: Smoothie Bowl (blend frozen berries, banana, spinach, Greek yogurt, and almond milk) topped with granola and sliced fruit.

- Lunch: Chickpea Salad with Feta, Cherry Tomatoes, Cucumber, and Balsamic Vinaigrette.
- Dinner: Turkey Meatballs (made with lean ground turkey, breadcrumbs, herbs) served with marinara sauce and zucchini noodles.

Day 5:

- Breakfast: Avocado Toast (whole grain toast topped with mashed avocado, sliced tomatoes, and a sprinkle of salt and pepper).
- Lunch: Spinach and Mushroom Stuffed Portobello Mushrooms served with a side of quinoa.
- Dinner: Vegetable Curry (potatoes, carrots, cauliflower, peas simmered in coconut milk and curry spices) served with brown rice.

Day 6:

- Breakfast: Scrambled Eggs with Spinach, Mushrooms, and Feta served with whole grain toast.
- Lunch: Quinoa Salad with Roasted Vegetables (such as bell peppers, zucchini, eggplant) and Lemon-Tahini Dressing.
- Dinner: Baked Chicken Breast with Rosemary and Garlic served with roasted sweet potatoes and green beans.

Day 7:

- Breakfast: Overnight Oats (combine rolled oats, almond milk, Greek yogurt, chia seeds, and sliced bananas) topped with nuts and honey.
- Lunch: Lentil Soup with Kale and Carrots served with a side of whole grain bread.

- Dinner: Grilled Salmon with Lemon-Dill Marinade served with quinoa and steamed asparagus.

Day 8:

- Breakfast: Greek Yogurt with Mixed Berries and Honey.
- Lunch: Chickpea and Vegetable Stir-Fry (chickpeas, bell peppers, broccoli, carrots) served with brown rice.
- Dinner: Turkey Chili (lean ground turkey, kidney beans, diced tomatoes, chili spices) served with a side of steamed green beans.

Day 9:

- Breakfast: Spinach and Feta Frittata (eggs, spinach, feta cheese) served with whole grain toast.
- Lunch: Quinoa Salad with Roasted Vegetables (such as sweet potatoes,

Brussels sprouts, and cauliflower) and Lemon-Tahini Dressing.

- Dinner: Baked Cod with Lemon-Herb Crust served with quinoa and steamed broccoli.

Day 10:

- Breakfast: Banana Almond Butter Smoothie (banana, almond butter, spinach, almond milk) topped with granola.
- Lunch: Lentil Soup with Kale and Carrots served with a side of whole grain bread.
- Dinner: Grilled Chicken Skewers with Mediterranean Salad (cucumbers, tomatoes, red onions, olives, feta cheese) and tzatziki sauce.

Day 11:

- Breakfast: Overnight Chia Seed Pudding (chia seeds, almond milk, vanilla extract) topped with sliced strawberries and almonds.

- Lunch: Caprese Stuffed Portobello Mushrooms served with a side salad.
- Dinner: Beef and Broccoli Stir-Fry (thinly sliced beef, broccoli, garlic) served with brown rice.

Day 12:

- Breakfast: Avocado Toast with Smoked Salmon (whole grain toast, mashed avocado, smoked salmon, lemon juice).
- Lunch: Greek Salad with Chickpeas (mixed greens, cherry tomatoes, cucumber, red onion, feta cheese, olives) served with grilled chicken breast.
- Dinner: Vegetable Curry (potatoes, carrots, cauliflower, peas) served with quinoa or brown rice.

Day 13:

- Breakfast: Vegetable Omelette (eggs, bell peppers, spinach, onions) served with whole grain toast.
- Lunch: Quinoa Salad with Chickpeas, Cherry Tomatoes, Cucumber, and Lemon-Tahini Dressing.
- Dinner: Baked Salmon with Herbs (salmon fillets marinated with olive oil, dill, parsley, garlic, lemon) served with roasted sweet potatoes and steamed broccoli.

Day 14:

- Breakfast: Greek Yogurt Parfait (Greek yogurt layered with granola and mixed berries).
- Lunch: Lentil Soup with Spinach and Carrots served with a side of whole grain bread.

- Dinner: Vegetable Stir-Fry (assorted vegetables stir-fried with tofu or chicken) served with brown rice.

Day 15:

- Breakfast: Banana Oatmeal (oatmeal topped with sliced bananas, chopped nuts, and a drizzle of honey).
- Lunch: Caprese Stuffed Portobello Mushrooms served with a side salad.
- Dinner: Beef and Broccoli Stir-Fry (thinly sliced beef stir-fried with broccoli and garlic) served with quinoa.

Day 16:

- Breakfast: Greek Yogurt with Mixed Berries and Honey.
- Lunch: Chickpea Salad with Feta, Cherry Tomatoes, Cucumber, and Balsamic Vinaigrette.

- Dinner: Baked Cod with Lemon-Herb Crust served with roasted sweet potatoes and steamed green beans.

Day 17:

- Breakfast: Spinach and Feta Frittata (eggs, spinach, feta cheese) served with whole grain toast.
- Lunch: Lentil Soup with Kale and Carrots served with a side of whole grain bread.
- Dinner: Grilled Chicken Skewers with Mediterranean Salad (cucumbers, tomatoes, red onions, olives, feta cheese) and tzatziki sauce.

Day 18:

- Breakfast: Avocado Toast with Smoked Salmon (whole grain toast, mashed avocado, smoked salmon, lemon juice).

- Lunch: Greek Salad with Chickpeas (mixed greens, cherry tomatoes, cucumber, red onion, feta cheese, olives) served with grilled chicken breast.
- Dinner: Vegetable Curry (potatoes, carrots, cauliflower, peas) served with quinoa or brown rice.

Day 19:

- Breakfast: Overnight Chia Seed Pudding (chia seeds, almond milk, vanilla extract) topped with sliced strawberries and almonds.
- Lunch: Quinoa Salad with Roasted Vegetables (such as sweet potatoes, Brussels sprouts, and cauliflower) and Lemon-Tahini Dressing.
- Dinner: Baked Salmon with Herbs (salmon fillets marinated with olive oil, dill, parsley, garlic, lemon) served with steamed broccoli and brown rice.

Day 20:

- Breakfast: Vegetable Omelette (eggs, bell peppers, spinach, onions) served with whole grain toast.
- Lunch: Quinoa Salad with Chickpeas, Cherry Tomatoes, Cucumber, and Lemon-Tahini Dressing.
- Dinner: Turkey Chili (lean ground turkey, kidney beans, diced tomatoes, chili spices) served with a side of steamed green beans.

Day 21:

- Breakfast: Banana Almond Butter Smoothie (banana, almond butter, spinach, almond milk) topped with granola.
- Lunch: Lentil Soup with Spinach and Carrots served with a side of whole grain bread.
- Dinner: Grilled Chicken Breast with Rosemary and Garlic served with

roasted sweet potatoes and steamed asparagus.

Day 22:

- Breakfast: Greek Yogurt Parfait (Greek yogurt layered with granola and mixed berries).
- Lunch: Lentil Soup with Spinach and Carrots served with a side of whole grain bread.
- Dinner: Vegetable Stir-Fry (assorted vegetables stir-fried with tofu or chicken) served with brown rice.

Day 23:

- Breakfast: Banana Oatmeal (oatmeal topped with sliced bananas, chopped nuts, and a drizzle of honey).
- Lunch: Caprese Stuffed Portobello Mushrooms served with a side salad.
- Dinner: Beef and Broccoli Stir-Fry (thinly sliced beef stir-fried with

broccoli and garlic) served with quinoa.

Day 24:

- Breakfast: Avocado Toast with Smoked Salmon (whole grain toast, mashed avocado, smoked salmon, lemon juice).
- Lunch: Greek Salad with Chickpeas (mixed greens, cherry tomatoes, cucumber, red onion, feta cheese, olives) served with grilled chicken breast.
- Dinner: Vegetable Curry (potatoes, carrots, cauliflower, peas) served with quinoa or brown rice.

Day 25:

- Breakfast: Spinach and Feta Frittata (eggs, spinach, feta cheese) served with whole grain toast.

- Lunch: Quinoa Salad with Roasted Vegetables (such as sweet potatoes, Brussels sprouts, and cauliflower) and Lemon-Tahini Dressing.
- Dinner: Baked Salmon with Lemon-Herb Crust served with roasted sweet potatoes and steamed green beans.

Day 26:

- Breakfast: Overnight Chia Seed Pudding (chia seeds, almond milk, vanilla extract) topped with sliced strawberries and almonds.
- Lunch: Chickpea Salad with Feta, Cherry Tomatoes, Cucumber, and Balsamic Vinaigrette.
- Dinner: Baked Cod with Lemon-Herb Crust served with roasted root vegetables and steamed asparagus.

Day 27:

- Breakfast: Vegetable Omelette (eggs, bell peppers, spinach, onions) served with whole grain toast.
- Lunch: Quinoa Salad with Chickpeas, Cherry Tomatoes, Cucumber, and Lemon-Tahini Dressing.
- Dinner: Turkey Chili (lean ground turkey, kidney beans, diced tomatoes, chili spices) served with a side of steamed green beans.

Day 28:

- Breakfast: Banana Almond Butter Smoothie (banana, almond butter, spinach, almond milk) topped with granola.
- Lunch: Lentil Soup with Spinach and Carrots served with a side of whole grain bread.
- Dinner: Grilled Chicken Skewers with Mediterranean Salad (cucumbers,

tomatoes, red onions, olives, feta cheese) and tzatziki sauce.

CONCLUSION

"Congratulations on taking the first step towards managing Parkinson's disease through nutrition! The Quick and Easy Complete Solution Parkinson's Disease Diet Cookbook for Beginners is more than just a cookbook - it's a comprehensive guide to empowering your health and well-being.

By incorporating the recipes and principles outlined in this book, you'll be taking control of your diet and nutrition, and making a positive impact on your overall health. Remember, every small change adds up, and the power of nutrition should not be underestimated.

Don't let Parkinson's disease hold you back - take charge of your health today! With this cookbook, you'll have the tools and confidence to cook delicious, nutritious meals that support your journey towards wellness.

Bon appétit, and remember to always prioritize your health and happiness!"

This conclusion aims to:

- Congratulate the reader on taking the first step towards managing Parkinson's disease through nutrition
- Emphasize the importance of empowerment and taking control of one's health
- Encourage the reader to continue making positive changes
- Offer support and motivation for their journey towards wellness
- End with a positive and uplifting note

THE END